My Essential Oil Recipes

a blank recipe book for <u>your</u> recipes & records

Thank you for your purchase!

This blank recipe book is intended as place to record your blends of oils and keep recipes you love from all other places.
You will also notice that there are areas to record each family members results to the recipe. This is great for reference.

At the back of the book you will find a list of essential oils.
I hope this helps you track your inventory.

Recipes Index

pg	Recipe	Condition	Diffuse	External	Internal
10					
11					
12					
13					
14					
15					
16					
17					
18					
19					
20					
21					
22					
23					
24					
25					
26					

pg	Recipe	Condition	⚕	💧	👤
27					
28					
29					
30					
31					
34					
35					
36					
37					
38					
39					
40					
41					
42					
43					
44					
45					
46					

pg	Recipe	Condition	🎋	💧	🗣
47					
48					
49					
50					
51					
54					
55					
56					
57					
58					
59					
60					
61					
62					
63					
64					
65					
66					

pg	Recipe	Condition	〰	💧	👤
67					
68					
69					
70					
71					
74					
75					
76					
77					
78					
79					
80					
81					
82					
83					
84					
85					
86					

pg	Recipe	Condition	ఇ	✍	🗣
87					
88					
89					
90					
91					
94					
95					
96					
97					
98					
99					
100					
101					
102					
103					
104					
105					
106					

pg	Recipe	Condition	🌀	💧	👤
107					
108					
109					
110					
111					
114					
115					
116					
117					
118					
119					
120					
121					
122					
123					
124					
125					
126					

pg	Recipe	Condition	🌀	💧	👤
127					
128					
129					
130					
131					
134					
135					
136					
137					
138					
139					
140					
141					
142					
143					
144					
145					
146					

pg	Recipe	Condition	৭৷৷৷	💧	🗣
147					

How to fill in a Recipe (Sample)

Recipe Name: Lavender & Citrus Freshener

1 tsp	vodka
15 drops	lavender essential oil
10 drops	grapefruit essential oil
500 ml	water

Uses: Mix together the vodka and essential oils in a 500ml spray bottle and shake well. Add water and shake again. Spray a fine mist into the air. Avoid spraying directly on fabrics or wood surfaces.

Family Results Record:

Date	Family Member	Condition	Application	Result
24 Apr	Joey	hyper	air	calming

Recipe Name:

Uses:

*

Family Results Record:

Date	Family Member	Condition	Application	Result

Recipe Name:

Uses:

Family Results Record:

Date	Family Member	Condition	Application	Result

Recipe Name:

Uses:

Family Results Record:

Date	Family Member	Condition	Application	Result

Recipe Name:

Uses:

Family Results Record:

Date	Family Member	Condition	Application	Result

Recipe Name:

Uses:

Family Results Record:

Date	Family Member	Condition	Application	Result

Recipe Name:

Uses:

Family Results Record:

Date	Family Member	Condition	Application	Result

Recipe Name:

Uses:

Family Results Record:

Date	Family Member	Condition	Application	Result

Recipe Name:

Uses:

Family Results Record:

Date	Family Member	Condition	Application	Result

Recipe Name:

Uses:

Family Results Record:

Date	Family Member	Condition	Application	Result

Recipe Name:

Uses:

Family Results Record:

Date	Family Member	Condition	Application	Result

Recipe Name:

_____

Uses:

_____

Family Results Record:

Date	Family Member	Condition	Application	Result

Recipe Name:

_____

Uses:

_____

Family Results Record:

Date	Family Member	Condition	Application	Result

Recipe Name:

Uses:

Family Results Record:

Date	Family Member	Condition	Application	Result

Recipe Name:

Uses:

Family Results Record:

Date	Family Member	Condition	Application	Result

Recipe Name:

Uses:

Family Results Record:

Date	Family Member	Condition	Application	Result

Recipe Name:

Uses:

Family Results Record:

Date	Family Member	Condition	Application	Result

Recipe Name:

Uses:

Family Results Record:

Date	Family Member	Condition	Application	Result

Recipe Name:

Uses:

Family Results Record:

Date	Family Member	Condition	Application	Result

Recipe Name:

Uses:

Family Results Record:

Date	Family Member	Condition	Application	Result

Recipe Name:

Uses:

Family Results Record:

Date	Family Member	Condition	Application	Result

Recipe Name:

Uses:

Family Results Record:

Date	Family Member	Condition	Application	Result

Recipe Name:

Uses:

Family Results Record:

Date	Family Member	Condition	Application	Result

Recipe Name:

Uses:

Family Results Record:

Date	Family Member	Condition	Application	Result

Recipe Name:

Uses:

Family Results Record:

Date	Family Member	Condition	Application	Result

Recipe Name:

Uses:

Family Results Record:

Date	Family Member	Condition	Application	Result

Recipe Name:

Uses:

Family Results Record:

Date	Family Member	Condition	Application	Result

Recipe Name:

Uses:

Family Results Record:

Date	Family Member	Condition	Application	Result

Recipe Name:

Uses:

Family Results Record:

Date	Family Member	Condition	Application	Result

Recipe Name:

Uses:

Family Results Record:

Date	Family Member	Condition	Application	Result

Recipe Name:

Uses:

Family Results Record:

Date	Family Member	Condition	Application	Result

Recipe Name:

Uses:

Family Results Record:

Date	Family Member	Condition	Application	Result

Recipe Name:

Uses:

Family Results Record:

Date	Family Member	Condition	Application	Result

Recipe Name:

Uses:

Family Results Record:

Date	Family Member	Condition	Application	Result

Recipe Name:

Uses:

Family Results Record:

Date	Family Member	Condition	Application	Result

Recipe Name:

Uses:

Family Results Record:

Date	Family Member	Condition	Application	Result

Recipe Name:

Uses:

Family Results Record:

Date	Family Member	Condition	Application	Result

Recipe Name:

Uses:

Family Results Record:

Date	Family Member	Condition	Application	Result

Recipe Name:

Uses:

Family Results Record:

Date	Family Member	Condition	Application	Result

Recipe Name:

Uses:

Family Results Record:

Date	Family Member	Condition	Application	Result

Recipe Name:

Uses:

Family Results Record:

Date	Family Member	Condition	Application	Result

Recipe Name:

Uses:

Family Results Record:

Date	Family Member	Condition	Application	Result

Recipe Name:

Uses:

Family Results Record:

Date	Family Member	Condition	Application	Result

Recipe Name:

Uses:

Family Results Record:

Date	Family Member	Condition	Application	Result

Recipe Name:

Uses:

Family Results Record:

Date	Family Member	Condition	Application	Result

Lavender

allergies
insomnia
anxiety
cold sores
burns
dandruff
yeast infections
ringworm
rash
and more

Recipe Name:

Uses:

Family Results Record:

Date	Family Member	Condition	Application	Result

Recipe Name:

Uses:

Family Results Record:

Date	Family Member	Condition	Application	Result

Recipe Name:

Uses:

Family Results Record:

Date	Family Member	Condition	Application	Result

Recipe Name:

Uses:

Family Results Record:

Date	Family Member	Condition	Application	Result

Recipe Name:

Uses:

Family Results Record:

Date	Family Member	Condition	Application	Result

Recipe Name:

Uses:

Family Results Record:

Date	Family Member	Condition	Application	Result

Recipe Name:

Uses:

Family Results Record:

Date	Family Member	Condition	Application	Result

Recipe Name:

Uses:

Family Results Record:

Date	Family Member	Condition	Application	Result

Recipe Name:

Uses:

Family Results Record:

Date	Family Member	Condition	Application	Result

Recipe Name:

Uses:

Family Results Record:

Date	Family Member	Condition	Application	Result

Recipe Name:

Uses:

Family Results Record:

Date	Family Member	Condition	Application	Result

Recipe Name:

Uses:

Family Results Record:

Date	Family Member	Condition	Application	Result

Recipe Name:

Uses:

Family Results Record:

Date	Family Member	Condition	Application	Result

Recipe Name:

Uses:

Family Results Record:

Date	Family Member	Condition	Application	Result

Recipe Name:

Uses:

Family Results Record:

Date	Family Member	Condition	Application	Result

Recipe Name:

Uses:

Family Results Record:

Date	Family Member	Condition	Application	Result

Recipe Name:

Uses:

Family Results Record:

Date	Family Member	Condition	Application	Result

Recipe Name:

Uses:

Family Results Record:

Date	Family Member	Condition	Application	Result

Recipe Name:

Uses:

Family Results Record:

Date	Family Member	Condition	Application	Result

Recipe Name:

Uses:

Family Results Record:

Date	Family Member	Condition	Application	Result

Recipe Name:

Uses:

Family Results Record:

Date	Family Member	Condition	Application	Result

Recipe Name:

Uses:

Family Results Record:

Date	Family Member	Condition	Application	Result

Recipe Name:

Uses:

Family Results Record:

Date	Family Member	Condition	Application	Result

Recipe Name:

Uses:

Family Results Record:

Date	Family Member	Condition	Application	Result

Recipe Name:

Uses:

Family Results Record:

Date	Family Member	Condition	Application	Result

Recipe Name:

Uses:

Family Results Record:

Date	Family Member	Condition	Application	Result

Recipe Name:

Uses:

Family Results Record:

Date	Family Member	Condition	Application	Result

Recipe Name:

Uses:

Family Results Record:

Date	Family Member	Condition	Application	Result

Recipe Name:

Uses:

Family Results Record:

Date	Family Member	Condition	Application	Result

Recipe Name:

Uses:

Family Results Record:

Date	Family Member	Condition	Application	Result

Recipe Name:

Uses:

Family Results Record:

Date	Family Member	Condition	Application	Result

Recipe Name:

Uses:

Family Results Record:

Date	Family Member	Condition	Application	Result

Recipe Name:

Uses:

Family Results Record:

Date	Family Member	Condition	Application	Result

Recipe Name:

Uses:

Family Results Record:

Date	Family Member	Condition	Application	Result

Recipe Name:

Uses:

Family Results Record:

Date	Family Member	Condition	Application	Result

Recipe Name:

Uses:

Family Results Record:

Date	Family Member	Condition	Application	Result

Lemon

uplifting aroma - excellent for moods
great to use to clean your home
and more

Recipe Name:

Uses:

Family Results Record:

Date	Family Member	Condition	Application	Result

Recipe Name:

Uses:

Family Results Record:

Date	Family Member	Condition	Application	Result

Recipe Name:

_____

Uses:

_____

Family Results Record:

Date	Family Member	Condition	Application	Result

Recipe Name:

_____

Uses:

_____

Family Results Record:

Date	Family Member	Condition	Application	Result

Recipe Name:

Uses:

Family Results Record:

Date	Family Member	Condition	Application	Result

Recipe Name:

Uses:

Family Results Record:

Date	Family Member	Condition	Application	Result

Recipe Name:

Uses:

Family Results Record:

Date	Family Member	Condition	Application	Result

Recipe Name:

Uses:

Family Results Record:

Date	Family Member	Condition	Application	Result

Recipe Name:

Uses:

Family Results Record:

Date	Family Member	Condition	Application	Result

Recipe Name:

Uses:

Family Results Record:

Date	Family Member	Condition	Application	Result

Recipe Name:

Uses:

Family Results Record:

Date	Family Member	Condition	Application	Result

Recipe Name:

Uses:

Family Results Record:

Date	Family Member	Condition	Application	Result

Recipe Name:

Uses:

Family Results Record:

Date	Family Member	Condition	Application	Result

Recipe Name:

Uses:

Family Results Record:

Date	Family Member	Condition	Application	Result

Recipe Name:

Uses:

Family Results Record:

Date	Family Member	Condition	Application	Result

Recipe Name:

Uses:

Family Results Record:

Date	Family Member	Condition	Application	Result

Recipe Name:

Uses:

Family Results Record:

Date	Family Member	Condition	Application	Result

Recipe Name:

Uses:

Family Results Record:

Date	Family Member	Condition	Application	Result

Recipe Name:

Uses:

Family Results Record:

Date	Family Member	Condition	Application	Result

Recipe Name:

Uses:

Family Results Record:

Date	Family Member	Condition	Application	Result

Recipe Name:

Uses:

Family Results Record:

Date	Family Member	Condition	Application	Result

Recipe Name:

Uses:

Family Results Record:

Date	Family Member	Condition	Application	Result

Recipe Name:

Uses:

Family Results Record:

Date	Family Member	Condition	Application	Result

Recipe Name:

Uses:

Family Results Record:

Date	Family Member	Condition	Application	Result

Recipe Name:

Uses:

Family Results Record:

Date	Family Member	Condition	Application	Result

Recipe Name:

Uses:

Family Results Record:

Date	Family Member	Condition	Application	Result

Recipe Name:

Uses:

Family Results Record:

Date	Family Member	Condition	Application	Result

Recipe Name:

Uses:

Family Results Record:

Date	Family Member	Condition	Application	Result

Recipe Name:

Uses:

Family Results Record:

Date	Family Member	Condition	Application	Result

Recipe Name:

Uses:

Family Results Record:

Date	Family Member	Condition	Application	Result

Recipe Name:

Uses:

Family Results Record:

Date	Family Member	Condition	Application	Result

Recipe Name:

Uses:

Family Results Record:

Date	Family Member	Condition	Application	Result

Recipe Name:

Uses:

Family Results Record:

Date	Family Member	Condition	Application	Result

Recipe Name:

Uses:

Family Results Record:

Date	Family Member	Condition	Application	Result

Recipe Name:

Uses:

Family Results Record:

Date	Family Member	Condition	Application	Result

Recipe Name:

Uses:

Family Results Record:

Date	Family Member	Condition	Application	Result

Peppermint

digestive tract
motion sickness
hearburn
headaches
itch
and more

Recipe Name:

Uses:

Family Results Record:

Date	Family Member	Condition	Application	Result

Recipe Name:

Uses:

Family Results Record:

Date	Family Member	Condition	Application	Result

Recipe Name:

Uses:

Family Results Record:

Date	Family Member	Condition	Application	Result

Recipe Name:

Uses:

Family Results Record:

Date	Family Member	Condition	Application	Result

Recipe Name:

Uses:

Family Results Record:

Date	Family Member	Condition	Application	Result

Recipe Name:

Uses:

Family Results Record:

Date	Family Member	Condition	Application	Result

Recipe Name:

Uses:

Family Results Record:

Date	Family Member	Condition	Application	Result

Recipe Name:

Uses:

Family Results Record:

Date	Family Member	Condition	Application	Result

Recipe Name:

Uses:

Family Results Record:

Date	Family Member	Condition	Application	Result

Recipe Name:

Uses:

Family Results Record:

Date	Family Member	Condition	Application	Result

Recipe Name:

Uses:

Family Results Record:

Date	Family Member	Condition	Application	Result

Recipe Name:

Uses:

Family Results Record:

Date	Family Member	Condition	Application	Result

Recipe Name:

Uses:

Family Results Record:

Date	Family Member	Condition	Application	Result

Recipe Name:

Uses:

Family Results Record:

Date	Family Member	Condition	Application	Result

Recipe Name:

Uses:

Family Results Record:

Date	Family Member	Condition	Application	Result

Recipe Name:

Uses:

Family Results Record:

Date	Family Member	Condition	Application	Result

Recipe Name:

Uses:

Family Results Record:

Date	Family Member	Condition	Application	Result

Recipe Name:

Uses:

Family Results Record:

Date	Family Member	Condition	Application	Result

Recipe Name:

Uses:

Family Results Record:

Date	Family Member	Condition	Application	Result

Recipe Name:

Uses:

Family Results Record:

Date	Family Member	Condition	Application	Result

Recipe Name:

Uses:

Family Results Record:

Date	Family Member	Condition	Application	Result

Recipe Name:

Uses:

Family Results Record:

Date	Family Member	Condition	Application	Result

Recipe Name:

Uses:

Family Results Record:

Date	Family Member	Condition	Application	Result

Recipe Name:

Uses:

Family Results Record:

Date	Family Member	Condition	Application	Result

Recipe Name:

Uses:

Family Results Record:

Date	Family Member	Condition	Application	Result

Recipe Name:

Uses:

Family Results Record:

Date	Family Member	Condition	Application	Result

Recipe Name:

Uses:

Family Results Record:

Date	Family Member	Condition	Application	Result

Recipe Name:

Uses:

Family Results Record:

Date	Family Member	Condition	Application	Result

Recipe Name:

Uses:

Family Results Record:

Date	Family Member	Condition	Application	Result

Recipe Name:

Uses:

Family Results Record:

Date	Family Member	Condition	Application	Result

Recipe Name:

Uses:

Family Results Record:

Date	Family Member	Condition	Application	Result

Recipe Name:

Uses:

Family Results Record:

Date	Family Member	Condition	Application	Result

Recipe Name:

Uses:

Family Results Record:

Date	Family Member	Condition	Application	Result

Recipe Name:

Uses:

Family Results Record:

Date	Family Member	Condition	Application	Result

Recipe Name:

Uses:

Family Results Record:

Date	Family Member	Condition	Application	Result

Recipe Name:

Uses:

Family Results Record:

Date	Family Member	Condition	Application	Result

Frankincense

healing support
depression
stretch marks / scars & skin care
and more

Recipe Name:

Uses:

Family Results Record:

Date	Family Member	Condition	Application	Result

Recipe Name:

Uses:

Family Results Record:

Date	Family Member	Condition	Application	Result

Recipe Name:

Uses:

Family Results Record:

Date	Family Member	Condition	Application	Result

Recipe Name:

Uses:

Family Results Record:

Date	Family Member	Condition	Application	Result

Recipe Name:

Uses:

Family Results Record:

Date	Family Member	Condition	Application	Result

Recipe Name:

Uses:

Family Results Record:

Date	Family Member	Condition	Application	Result

Recipe Name:

Uses:

Family Results Record:

Date	Family Member	Condition	Application	Result

Recipe Name:

Uses:

Family Results Record:

Date	Family Member	Condition	Application	Result

Recipe Name:

Uses:

Family Results Record:

Date	Family Member	Condition	Application	Result

Recipe Name:

Uses:

Family Results Record:

Date	Family Member	Condition	Application	Result

Recipe Name:

Uses:

Family Results Record:

Date	Family Member	Condition	Application	Result

Recipe Name:

Uses:

Family Results Record:

Date	Family Member	Condition	Application	Result

Recipe Name:

Uses:

Family Results Record:

Date	Family Member	Condition	Application	Result

Recipe Name:

Uses:

Family Results Record:

Date	Family Member	Condition	Application	Result

Recipe Name:

Uses:

Family Results Record:

Date	Family Member	Condition	Application	Result

Recipe Name:

Uses:

Family Results Record:

Date	Family Member	Condition	Application	Result

Recipe Name:

Uses:

Family Results Record:

Date	Family Member	Condition	Application	Result

Recipe Name:

Uses:

Family Results Record:

Date	Family Member	Condition	Application	Result

Recipe Name:

Uses:

Family Results Record:

Date	Family Member	Condition	Application	Result

Recipe Name:

Uses:

Family Results Record:

Date	Family Member	Condition	Application	Result

Recipe Name:

Uses:

Family Results Record:

Date	Family Member	Condition	Application	Result

Recipe Name:

Uses:

Family Results Record:

Date	Family Member	Condition	Application	Result

Recipe Name:

Uses:

Family Results Record:

Date	Family Member	Condition	Application	Result

Recipe Name:

Uses:

Family Results Record:

Date	Family Member	Condition	Application	Result

Recipe Name:

Uses:

Family Results Record:

Date	Family Member	Condition	Application	Result

Recipe Name:

Uses:

Family Results Record:

Date	Family Member	Condition	Application	Result

Recipe Name:

Uses:

Family Results Record:

Date	Family Member	Condition	Application	Result

Recipe Name:

Uses:

Family Results Record:

Date	Family Member	Condition	Application	Result

Recipe Name:

Uses:

Family Results Record:

Date	Family Member	Condition	Application	Result

Recipe Name:

Uses:

Family Results Record:

Date	Family Member	Condition	Application	Result

Recipe Name:

Uses:

Family Results Record:

Date	Family Member	Condition	Application	Result

Recipe Name:

Uses:

Family Results Record:

Date	Family Member	Condition	Application	Result

Recipe Name:

Uses:

Family Results Record:

Date	Family Member	Condition	Application	Result

Recipe Name:

Uses:

Family Results Record:

Date	Family Member	Condition	Application	Result

Recipe Name:

Uses:

Family Results Record:

Date	Family Member	Condition	Application	Result

Recipe Name:

Uses:

Family Results Record:

Date	Family Member	Condition	Application	Result

Eucalyptus

invigorating aroma
aids in colds
insect repellent
increase circulation
disinfectant
and more

Recipe Name:

Uses:

Family Results Record:

Date	Family Member	Condition	Application	Result

Recipe Name:

Uses:

Family Results Record:

Date	Family Member	Condition	Application	Result

Recipe Name:

Uses:

Family Results Record:

Date	Family Member	Condition	Application	Result

Recipe Name:

Uses:

Family Results Record:

Date	Family Member	Condition	Application	Result

Recipe Name:

Uses:

Family Results Record:

Date	Family Member	Condition	Application	Result

Recipe Name:

Uses:

Family Results Record:

Date	Family Member	Condition	Application	Result

Recipe Name:

Uses:

Family Results Record:

Date	Family Member	Condition	Application	Result

Recipe Name:

Uses:

Family Results Record:

Date	Family Member	Condition	Application	Result

Recipe Name:

Uses:

Family Results Record:

Date	Family Member	Condition	Application	Result

Recipe Name:

Uses:

Family Results Record:

Date	Family Member	Condition	Application	Result

Recipe Name:

Uses:

Family Results Record:

Date	Family Member	Condition	Application	Result

Recipe Name:

Uses:

Family Results Record:

Date	Family Member	Condition	Application	Result

Recipe Name:

Uses:

Family Results Record:

Date	Family Member	Condition	Application	Result

Recipe Name:

Uses:

Family Results Record:

Date	Family Member	Condition	Application	Result

Recipe Name:

Uses:

Family Results Record:

Date	Family Member	Condition	Application	Result

Recipe Name:

Uses:

Family Results Record:

Date	Family Member	Condition	Application	Result

Recipe Name:

Uses:

Family Results Record:

Date	Family Member	Condition	Application	Result

Recipe Name:

Uses:

Family Results Record:

Date	Family Member	Condition	Application	Result

Recipe Name:

Uses:

Family Results Record:

Date	Family Member	Condition	Application	Result

Recipe Name:

Uses:

Family Results Record:

Date	Family Member	Condition	Application	Result

Recipe Name:

Uses:

Family Results Record:

Date	Family Member	Condition	Application	Result

Recipe Name:

Uses:

Family Results Record:

Date	Family Member	Condition	Application	Result

Recipe Name:

Uses:

Family Results Record:

Date	Family Member	Condition	Application	Result

Recipe Name:

Uses:

Family Results Record:

Date	Family Member	Condition	Application	Result

Recipe Name: ＿＿＿＿＿＿＿＿＿＿＿＿＿＿＿＿＿＿＿＿＿＿＿＿＿＿＿＿＿＿＿

Uses:

Family Results Record:

Date	Family Member	Condition	Application	Result

Recipe Name: ＿＿＿＿＿＿＿＿＿＿＿＿＿＿＿＿＿＿＿＿＿＿＿＿＿＿＿＿＿＿＿

Uses:

Family Results Record:

Date	Family Member	Condition	Application	Result

Recipe Name:

Uses:

Family Results Record:

Date	Family Member	Condition	Application	Result

Recipe Name:

Uses:

Family Results Record:

Date	Family Member	Condition	Application	Result

Recipe Name:

Uses:

Family Results Record:

Date	Family Member	Condition	Application	Result

Recipe Name:

Uses:

Family Results Record:

Date	Family Member	Condition	Application	Result

Recipe Name:

Uses:

Family Results Record:

Date	Family Member	Condition	Application	Result

Recipe Name:

Uses:

Family Results Record:

Date	Family Member	Condition	Application	Result

Recipe Name:

Uses:

Family Results Record:

Date	Family Member	Condition	Application	Result

Recipe Name:

Uses:

Family Results Record:

Date	Family Member	Condition	Application	Result

Recipe Name:

Uses:

Family Results Record:

Date	Family Member	Condition	Application	Result

Recipe Name:

Uses:

Family Results Record:

Date	Family Member	Condition	Application	Result

Tea Tree

viral & bacterial infections
mouth infections
first aid kit must have
sunburn
toothpaste / deodorant
and more

Recipe Name:

Uses:

Family Results Record:

Date	Family Member	Condition	Application	Result

Recipe Name:

Uses:

Family Results Record:

Date	Family Member	Condition	Application	Result

Recipe Name:

Uses:

Family Results Record:

Date	Family Member	Condition	Application	Result

Recipe Name:

Uses:

Family Results Record:

Date	Family Member	Condition	Application	Result

Recipe Name:

Uses:

Family Results Record:

Date	Family Member	Condition	Application	Result

Recipe Name:

Uses:

Family Results Record:

Date	Family Member	Condition	Application	Result

Recipe Name:

Uses:

Family Results Record:

Date	Family Member	Condition	Application	Result

Recipe Name:

Uses:

Family Results Record:

Date	Family Member	Condition	Application	Result

Recipe Name:

Uses:

Family Results Record:

Date	Family Member	Condition	Application	Result

Recipe Name:

Uses:

Family Results Record:

Date	Family Member	Condition	Application	Result

Recipe Name:

Uses:

Family Results Record:

Date	Family Member	Condition	Application	Result

Recipe Name:

Uses:

Family Results Record:

Date	Family Member	Condition	Application	Result

Recipe Name:

Uses:

Family Results Record:

Date	Family Member	Condition	Application	Result

Recipe Name:

Uses:

Family Results Record:

Date	Family Member	Condition	Application	Result

Recipe Name:

Uses:

Family Results Record:

Date	Family Member	Condition	Application	Result

Recipe Name:

Uses:

Family Results Record:

Date	Family Member	Condition	Application	Result

Recipe Name:

Uses:

Family Results Record:

Date	Family Member	Condition	Application	Result

Recipe Name:

Uses:

Family Results Record:

Date	Family Member	Condition	Application	Result

Recipe Name:

Uses:

Family Results Record:

Date	Family Member	Condition	Application	Result

Recipe Name:

Uses:

Family Results Record:

Date	Family Member	Condition	Application	Result

Recipe Name:

Uses:

Family Results Record:

Date	Family Member	Condition	Application	Result

Recipe Name:

Uses:

Family Results Record:

Date	Family Member	Condition	Application	Result

Recipe Name:

Uses:

Family Results Record:

Date	Family Member	Condition	Application	Result

Recipe Name:

Uses:

Family Results Record:

Date	Family Member	Condition	Application	Result

Recipe Name:

Uses:

Family Results Record:

Date	Family Member	Condition	Application	Result

Recipe Name:

Uses:

Family Results Record:

Date	Family Member	Condition	Application	Result

Recipe Name:

Uses:

Family Results Record:

Date	Family Member	Condition	Application	Result

Recipe Name:

Uses:

Family Results Record:

Date	Family Member	Condition	Application	Result

My Essential Oil Stock

☐	Bergamot		☐		
☐	Cedarwood		☐		
☐	Cistus		☐		
☐	Citronella		☐		
☐	Clary Sage		☐		
☐	Clove		☐		
☐	Cypress		☐		
☐	Dill		☐		
☐	Eucalyptus		☐		
☐	Fennel		☐		
☐	Frankincense		☐		
☐	Ginger		☐		
☐	Grapefruit		☐		
☐	Jasmine		☐		
☐	Juniper		☐		
☐	Lavender		☐		
☐	Lemon		☐		
☐	Lemongrass		☐		
☐	Marjoram		☐		
☐	Melaleuca Alternifolia		☐		
☐	Melissa		☐		
☐	Neroli		☐		
☐	Orange		☐		
☐	Oregano		☐		
☐	Peppermint		☐		
☐	Pine		☐		
☐	Rose		☐		
☐	Rosemary		☐		
☐	Sage		☐		
☐	Sandalwood		☐		
☐	Spearmint		☐		
☐	Thyme		☐		
☐	Valerian		☐		
☐	Wintergreen		☐		
☐	Ylang Ylang		☐		

☐			☐		
☐			☐		
☐			☐		
☐			☐		
☐			☐		
☐			☐		
☐			☐		
☐			☐		
☐			☐		
☐			☐		
☐			☐		
☐			☐		
☐			☐		
☐			☐		
☐			☐		
☐			☐		
☐			☐		
☐			☐		
☐			☐		
☐			☐		
☐			☐		
☐			☐		
☐			☐		
☐			☐		
☐			☐		
☐			☐		
☐			☐		
☐			☐		
☐			☐		
☐			☐		
☐			☐		
☐			☐		
☐			☐		
☐			☐		
☐			☐		

☐			☐		
☐			☐		
☐			☐		
☐			☐		
☐			☐		
☐			☐		
☐			☐		
☐			☐		
☐			☐		
☐			☐		
☐			☐		
☐			☐		
☐			☐		
☐			☐		
☐			☐		
☐			☐		
☐			☐		
☐			☐		
☐			☐		
☐			☐		
☐			☐		
☐			☐		
☐			☐		
☐			☐		
☐			☐		
☐			☐		
☐			☐		
☐			☐		
☐			☐		
☐			☐		
☐			☐		
☐			☐		
☐			☐		
☐			☐		
☐			☐		
☐			☐		

60412603R00084

Made in the USA
Middletown, DE
29 December 2017